Bear Hugs for Being Healthy

*Positive activities that foster healthful
attitudes and behaviors*

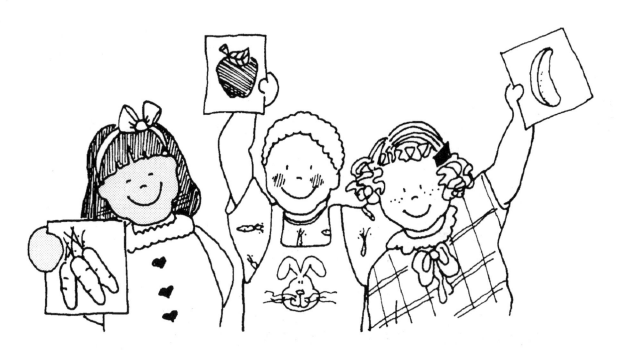

By Patty Claycomb and Gayle Bittinger
Illustrated by Marion Hopping Ekberg

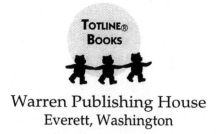

TOTLINE® BOOKS

Warren Publishing House
Everett, Washington

We wish to thank the following teachers for contributing some of the ideas in this book: Ellen Bedford, Bridgeport, CT; Janice Bodenstedt, Jackson, MI; Laurlie Mann, Hermosa Beach, CA; Paula Schneider, Kent, WA.

Editorial Staff
   Managing Editor: Kathleen Cubley
   Contributing Editors: Kate Ffolliott, Susan Hodges,
    Elizabeth McKinnon, Jean Warren
   Copy Editor: Mae Rhodes
   Proofreader: Kris Fulsaas

Design and Production Staff
   Art Managers: Uma Kukathas, Jill Lustig
   Book Design/Layout: Carol DeBolt, Sarah Ness
   Cover Design: Brenda Mann Harrison
   Digital Coloring: Sarah Ness
   Cover Illustration: Marion Hopping Ekberg
   Bear Hugs Logo: Susan Dahlman
   Production Manager: Jo Anna Brock

ISBN 1-57029-036-9

Printed in the United States of America
Published by: Warren Publishing House
            P.O. Box 2250
            Everett, WA 98203

20 19 18 17 16 15 14 13 12 11 10 9 8 7 6 5 4 3 2 1

Introduction

When germs and junk food start taking over your children's bodies, try some of these healthy Bear Hugs to get them back on the right track. Young children are so eager to learn about their bodies, and these activities help them do just that. From learning about germs and hand washing to healthy food choices, from exercising and resting their bodies to taking care of their teeth, this book has great ideas for instilling healthy attitudes and behaviors in your children.

Like the other books in the Bear Hugs series, *Bear Hugs for Being Healthy* provides you with simple, positive ideas that your children will love. Providing your children with information about ways they can keep themselves healthy and growing strong helps them feel great both inside and out.

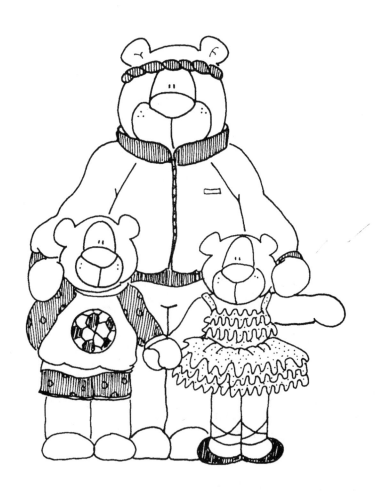

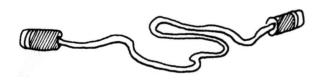

Contents

Sponge Toss

Encourage your children to develop good personal hygiene habits with this Bear Hug.

Materials: Sponge.

Preparation: None.

Activity: Have your children sit in a circle. Talk about the different ways that animals clean themselves. For example, cats clean themselves by licking their fur with their tongue, rabbits comb their ears and lick their paws, chickens "frazzle" themselves by shaking sand all over their ruffled feathers, beavers comb their fur with comblike claws, and bats clean themselves when they are hanging upside down.

Now discuss how humans clean themselves. Talk about activities such as washing hands, taking a bath, taking a shower, cleaning under fingernails, and washing hair. Next, play the Sponge Toss game. Gently toss the sponge to one of your children. Have the child say a way that people can clean themselves. Let that child gently toss the sponge to another child who then names another way to keep clean. Continue until each child has had a turn.

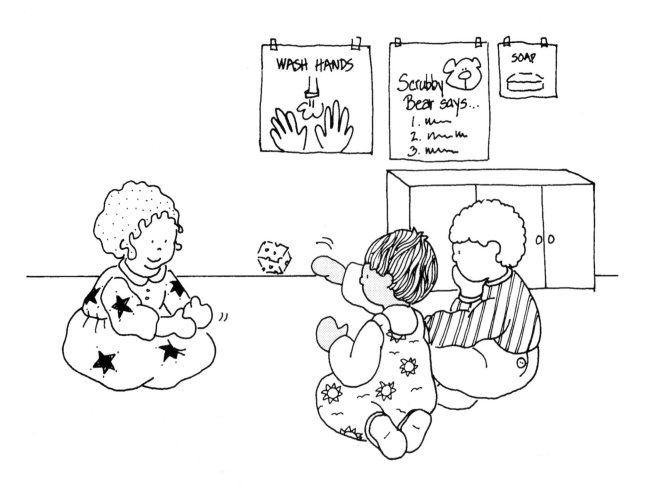

When Do You Wash Your Hands?

This Bear Hug will help your children learn when to wash their hands.

Materials: Construction paper; felt tip markers; scissors; wrapper from bar of soap; posterboard; tape.

Preparation: Cut the shape of a faucet and several hand shapes out of the construction paper. Write "We Wash Our Hands" across the top of the posterboard. Tape the faucet shape and the soap wrapper to the posterboard.

Activity: Show the posterboard to your children. Ask them what they do at a sink with water and soap. (Wash their hands.) Have them tell you the different times they should wash their hands. Possible answers include: before eating, after going to the bathroom, after petting an animal, when your hands get messy or sticky, after blowing your nose, and so on. After each response, sing the following song, substituting that response for *Before we go to eat our snack.*

> **Sung to: "The Farmer in the Dell"**
>
> **We will wash our hands.**
> **We will wash our hands.**
> **Before we go to eat our snack,**
> **We will wash our hands.**
>
> *Gayle Bittinger*

On each of the hand shapes, draw a simple picture to represent the different responses. Tape the hand shapes to the posterboard, underneath the faucet shape. Hang the posterboard by the sink to remind the children to wash their hands often.

Variation: Instead of drawing on the hand shapes, find appropriate magazine pictures to glue onto them.

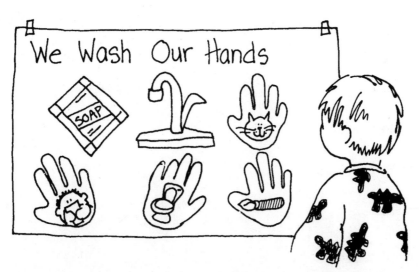

Hand-Washing Song

Use this musical Bear Hug to help your children remember how to effectively wash their hands.

Materials: None.

Preparation: None.

Activity: Talk with your children about the different steps involved in washing their hands. Emphasize the importance of all the steps: wetting hands, soaping them up, rinsing them, and drying them really well. Act out all the steps together. Then teach your children the following song to help them remember the steps. If you wish, substitute the name of your next activity, such as *snack* or *circle*, for the word *play*.

> **Sung to: "Jingle Bells"**
>
> **Wet your hands, soap your hands,**
> **Rub them to and fro.**
> **Rinse your hands and dry your hands,**
> **Then off to play you go.**
> **Wet your hands, soap your hands,**
> **Rub them to and fro.**
> **Rinse your hands and dry your hands,**
> **Then off to play you go.**
>
> *Ellen Bedford*

Extension: Make a picture chart with the steps illustrated and hang it by the sink.

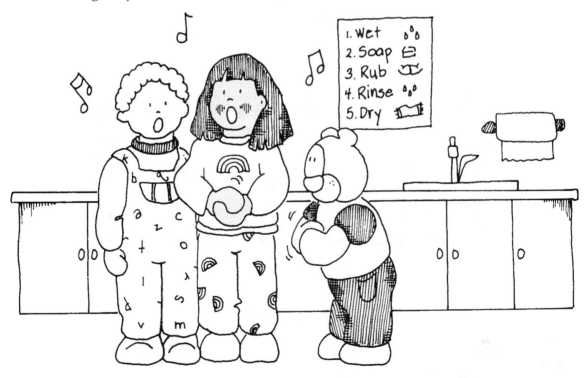

Shoulder Cough

This Bear Hug teaches your children a simple technique for covering their mouths while coughing.

Materials: Spray bottle; water.

Preparation: Fill the spray bottle with water.

Activity: Discuss coughing with your children and how it spreads germs. Demonstrate this for the children by using the spray bottle to squirt water into the air over their heads. Can they feel the droplets of water? Tell them that this is similar to what happens when they cough—tiny droplets of saliva filled with germs spray out of their mouths. When they land on other people, the germs can make those people sick. Tell the children this is why it is so important for them to cover their mouths when they cough. But what happens if they cough into their hands? (The germs get on their hands, and then they should wash them.)

Now tell your children you have a special way they can cough that keeps the germs out of the air and off their hands—the Shoulder Cough. Demonstrate this special cough by turning your head and placing your mouth on your raised arm and shoulder. Cough. All the germs are caught in your clothes. Have the children practice this technique. Read the following rhyme to the children. Encourage them to remind one another to do the Shoulder Cough.

> **When your throat just has a tickle,**
> **And you're feeling in a pickle,**
> **Don't forget to turn your head**
> **And do the Shoulder Cough instead.**
>
> *Gayle Bittinger*

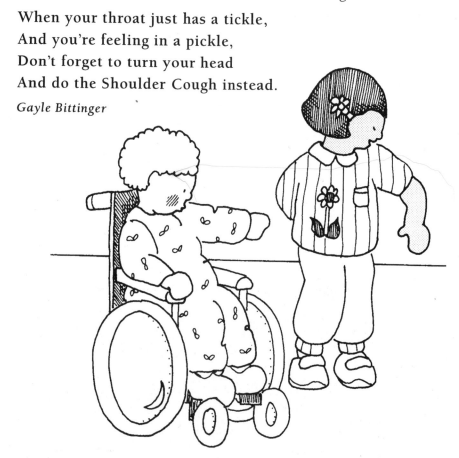

Tissue Time

*This Bear Hug will help your children remember what to do
after using a tissue.*

Materials: Paper; scissors; facial tissue box; pen; tape.

Preparation: Cut a piece of paper to fit on the front of the facial tissue box. Draw simple pictures of the following steps on the paper: using the tissue, dropping it in a garbage can, and washing hands. Tape the paper to the front of the box of tissues.

Activity: Show the tissue box to your children. Read the following rhyme to them.

> **After using this tissue,**
> **Please throw it away.**
> **Then go wash your hands**
> **Before you go play.**
>
> *Ellen Bedford*

Talk about the importance of throwing the tissue away, not leaving it on the table or floor or handing it to a teacher. Ask the children why it would also be important to wash their hands after blowing their nose. Encourage the idea that both of these steps help prevent germs from getting all around the classroom, making everyone sick.

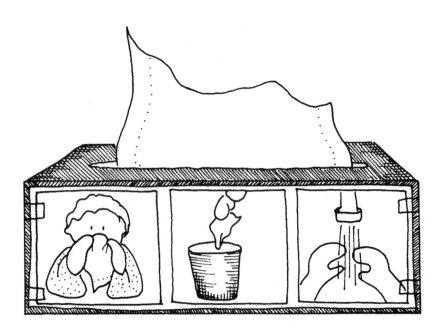

Time for Breakfast

Help your children understand the importance of eating a healthy breakfast with this Bear Hug.

Materials: Magazines; scissors; paper plates.

Preparation: Cut a variety of pictures of healthy breakfast foods, such as fruits, juices, toast, pancakes, and eggs, out of magazines.

Activity: Have your children lie down on the floor and pretend they are sleeping. Say "Time for breakfast," and have everyone wake up and get ready for "breakfast" by sitting in a circle. Place the pictures of food in the middle of the circle. One at a time, give each child a paper plate and let him or her choose one or two pictures to put on it. When all the children have been "served," sing the following song for each child, substituting the name of the child and his or her choice for *Ryan* and *orange juice*.

> **Sung to: "Mary Wore a Red Dress"**
>
> **Ryan's having orange juice,**
> **Orange juice, orange juice.**
> **Ryan's having orange juice**
> **For breakfast.**
>
> *Gayle Bittinger*

After the song, talk about why the foods they have chosen are good ones for starting out the day. (They provide energy and vitamins.)

Extension: In addition to the pictures and paper plate from the activity, give each of your children a sheet of construction paper and a napkin. Have them glue their napkin and paper plate to the construction paper, and the food pictures to the plate. Let them take home this reminder to eat a healthy breakfast.

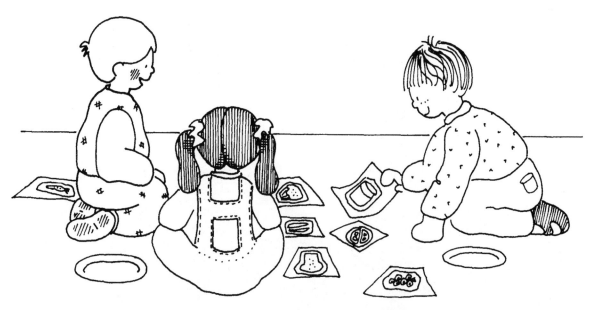

Healthy Shopping

Let your children practice making food selections with this Bear Hug.

Materials: Bookshelf or table; selection of grocery items, such as toy foods and empty food containers (be sure to include healthy and not-so-healthy choices); child-size shopping cart, wagon, or grocery bag with handles.

Preparation: Arrange the grocery items on the bookshelf or table.

Activity: Invite one of your children to go grocery shopping. Let the child select ten items to put into the shopping cart. Have the child bring the selections to you so you can "ring them up." Talk with the child about the choices he or she has made. Which foods are healthy? Which ones are not? Which ones will help the child grow big and strong? Let the child go shopping one more time. This time, ask him or her to choose only healthy foods. Continue throughout the week until each child has had a chance to go shopping.

Extension: Set up a shopping area in your dramatic play corner. Let your children take turns shopping and being the cashier. Encourage them to talk to one another about which foods are healthy and which ones are not.

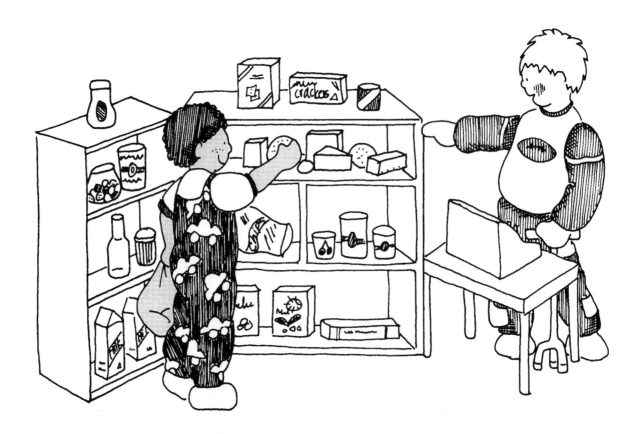

Food Pyramid

Use this easy Bear Hug to teach your children about which food choices are the best.

Materials: Two 6-foot lengths of butcher paper; tape; felt tip marker; magazines; scissors; glue.

Preparation: Tape the long sides of the butcher paper together. Place the paper on the floor. Draw a large triangle on the paper, divide it into sections, and label the sections as shown in the illustration to make a Food Pyramid. Cut out magazine pictures to represent the following food groups: grains, fruits, vegetables, dairy, protein, and fats and sweets. Cut out a number of pictures for each food group. The number will vary, depending on how large each space is on the Food Pyramid.

Activity: Show your children the pictures of food. Ask them to help you sort the pictures according to the kind of food they are. Have them glue the pictures in the appropriate spaces on the Food Pyramid. Explain that the foods they see the most of are the foods they should eat the most. Help them to think about this by asking them these questions: Should you eat more bread or more eggs? Should you eat more apples or more candy bars? Should you eat more carrots or more cheese? Encourage them to talk about the foods they eat and where those foods would go on the Food Pyramid.

Sung to: "If You're Happy and You Know It"

Oh, this pyramid is filled with food.
It shows us how to eat as we should.
This pyramid, you see,
Has food that's good for me.
Oh, this pyramid is filled with food.

Gayle Bittinger

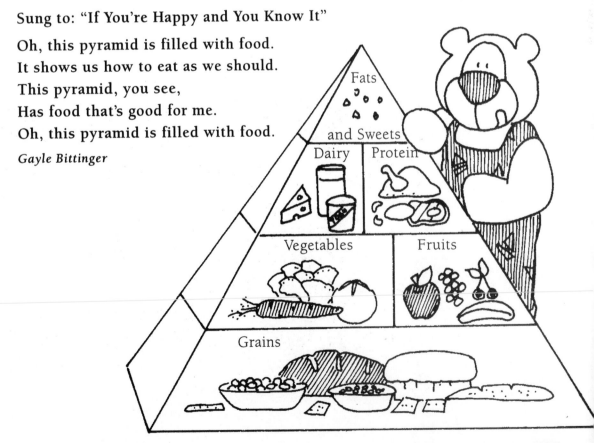

Food Helps Us Grow

Explain to your children why we eat and how food helps us with this Bear Hug.

Materials: None.

Preparation: None.

Activity: Have your children sit in a circle. Talk with them about why people need to eat. Use questions such as the following to foster your discussion: What should you do when your body is hungry? Could you eat just once a week? How does your body get energy for working and playing? How do you feel if you eat too much? Too little? Too many sweets? How does your body grow up healthy and strong?

Explain that all bodies need healthy food to grow. Have the children lie on the floor and pretend they are babies. Tell them that babies drink their food—milk—and that milk gives them energy to grow. Now have the children pretend they are toddlers and walk around the floor on their knees. Does food help toddlers grow? (Yes.) Next have the children stand up straight and tall and be themselves. Does food help them grow? (Of course.) Finally, have the children stand on their tiptoes and pretend to be older. Is food still helping them grow? (Absolutely.) Encourage the idea that eating healthy food will help them grow healthy and strong, and then sing the following song with them.

Sung to: "Row, Row, Row Your Boat"

Food, food helps us grow,
Helps us grow so strong.
Healthy food is what we need
So we can move along.

Food, food helps us grow.
Food helps you and me.
When we eat healthy food,
We're filled with energy!

Jean Warren

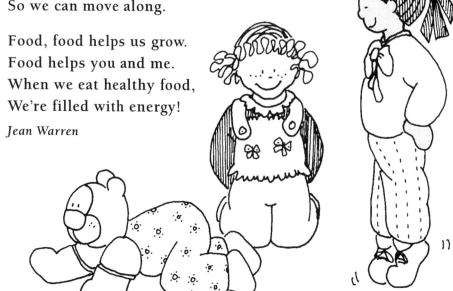

How Does Your Body Grow?

Help your children understand some of the things they need for their bodies to grow strong and healthy.

Materials: Magazines; scissors; construction paper; glue.

Preparation: From magazines, cut pictures of healthy foods, healthy drinks (including water), and children and adults being active. Glue each picture to a separate sheet of construction paper.

Activity: Have your children tell you the things their bodies need to grow strong and healthy. Encourage the idea that their bodies need healthy food to eat, liquids to drink, and exercise. Divide your children into three groups. Give to one group the pictures of healthy foods, to another group the pictures of healthy drinks, and to the third group the pictures of active people. Recite the rhyme below. Have the children hold up their pictures as they are mentioned in the rhyme.

Mary, Mary, quite contrary,
How does your body grow?
With healthy apples and carrots and bread,
And other foods, I know.

Mary, Mary, quite contrary,
How does your body grow?
With lots of water and juice and milk,
And other drinks, I know.

Mary, Mary, quite contrary,
How does your body grow?
With playing and moving all around
For exercise, I know.

Jean Warren

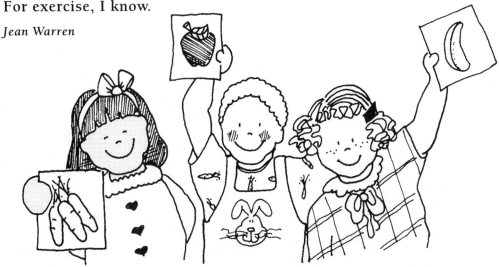

Heartbeats

This Bear Hug will help your children become familiar with exercise and how it helps their heart grow strong.

Materials: None.

Preparation: None.

Activity: Ask your children to show you where their heart is. Have them place their hands over their heart. Tell them that their heart is a muscle, just like the muscles in their arms and legs. Explain that the heart's job is to pump blood all over their body. Show the children how to clasp their hands together. Say "lub-dub, lub-dub, lub-dub" slowly and have the children squeeze and release their clasped hands to imitate the heart's pumping.

Discuss how exercise makes their heart muscle strong. Tell the children that when they exercise, their heart pumps faster. Have the children clasp their hands again. Say "lub-dub, lub-lub, lub-dub" again, only faster. Have the children squeeze and release their hands to the beat. Tell them this is how their heart works when they are exercising.

Now have the children exercise their heart and make it beat faster. Have them do some jumping jacks, jog in place, or, if possible, run around outside. When they are through, have them sit quietly and place a hand over their heart. Can they feel their heart pumping? Explain that if they can, they have exercised their heart and are making it strong. Tell them that they should try to exercise their heart at least once a day.

Variation: Bring in a stethoscope. Let your children take turns listening to their heart before and after exercising.

Extension: Draw a simple outline of a real heart on a sheet of paper. Make a copy of the drawing for each of your children. Let the children color the heart. Give them heart stickers to put on their heart as a reminder to love and take care of it.

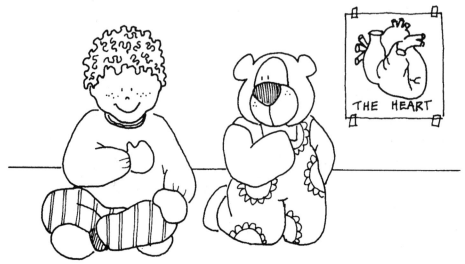

THE HEART

Exercising Game

Let your children have fun exercising and counting with this Bear Hug.

Materials: Index cards; felt tip markers.

Preparation: Draw simple pictures of exercises on several index cards. Include exercises such as toe touches, jogging in place, jumping jacks, and arm circles. Number ten additional index cards from 1 to 10. Mix up the exercise cards and place them in a pile. Repeat with the number cards.

Activity: Tell your children that it's time to exercise and you will need their help to choose which exercises and how many of each they should do. Have one child select one of the exercise cards and help the child name the exercise pictured on it. Have another child select one of the number cards and help him or her say the number on it. Then do the exercise that number of times while you sing the following song. Substitute the appropriate exercise and number for those in the song.

> **Sung to: "Skip to My Lou"**
>
> **Touch your toes seven times,**
> **Touch your toes seven times,**
> **Touch your toes seven times,**
> **To keep your body healthy.**
>
> *Gayle Bittinger*

Put the cards back in their respective piles. Then let two more children select cards. Repeat until each child has had a chance to select at least one card.

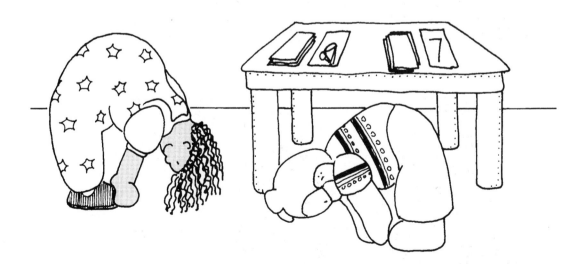

Sleep Tight

*Your children will understand the need for proper rest
with this sleepy Bear Hug.*

Materials: None.

Preparation: None.

Activity: Talk with your children about why it is important to rest their bodies and get plenty of sleep. Act out the following scene with them. Have the children jog in place, and then ask them to sit down. Talk about what a long day it has been and how much work they have done. Then have them pretend to go to bed. But instead of sleeping, ask them to play all night long. Now say, "Good morning!" and have the children get out of bed. Talk about how tired their bodies feel. Have them pretend to be exhausted while they try to get dressed, eat, and brush their teeth. They are so tired they can hardly move.

Ask the children what happens to their body when they don't get enough sleep. Explain that they just don't have the energy to do anything. Now act out getting a good night's sleep. Have the children wake up with lots of energy for getting dressed, eating breakfast, brushing teeth, and going to school. Encourage the idea that resting and letting their body sleep at night means their body will feel healthier and stronger the next day. Finish by reading the following rhyme to the children.

> **There's a time to sit and a time to play,**
> **And there's a time to run around all day.**
> **But when the night begins to come,**
> **And all your busy work is done,**
> **Plump your pillow in a heap**
> **And quietly go to sleep.**
>
> *Patty Claycomb*

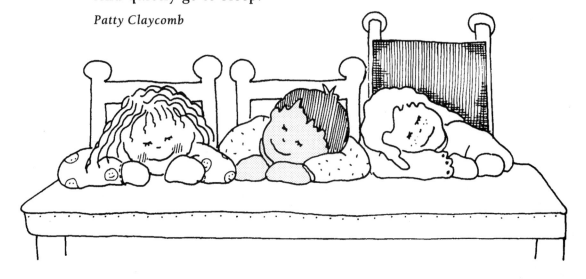

Brush Your Teeth

Teach your children proper brushing technique with this Bear Hug.

Materials: Heavy paper; felt tip marker; toothbrush.

Preparation: On the heavy paper, draw a big, open, smiley face with lots of teeth and a tongue.

Activity: Discuss with your children why we need to brush our teeth. Explain that after we eat, tiny cavity germs (bacteria) get on our teeth. The germs like to nibble on the surface of the teeth and make them sick. Ask them how they can get rid of the cavity germs. (Brush their teeth really well.) Show the children the smiley face. Demonstrate the "wiggle-jiggle" technique for brushing teeth by moving the brush in little circles at the gumline of each tooth. Tell the children to be sure to brush their tongue also because that is where many cavity germs "hide" after their teeth have been brushed. Sing the following song while you brush the tooth drawing.

> **Sung to: "If You're Happy and You Know It"**
>
> **When you want to brush your teeth—wiggle-jiggle.**
> **When you want to brush your teeth—wiggle-jiggle.**
> **First you wiggle, then you jiggle,**
> **Then brush your tongue until you giggle.**
> **When you want to brush your teeth—wiggle-jiggle.**
>
> *Gayle Bittinger*

Variation: Instead of showing your children how to brush teeth drawn on paper, ask your dentist if he or she has a set of practice teeth you could borrow for your demonstration.

Extension: Give each of your children a toothbrush and help them individually with their brushing technique.

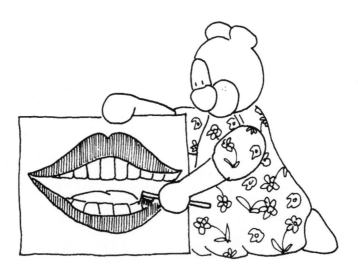

Happy Teeth

Help your children understand ways to keep their teeth healthy with this Bear Hug.

Materials: Red and white construction paper; scissors; glue.

Preparation: For each child, cut a 6- by 4-inch smiling lips shape out of the red construction paper and a 1/2- by 8-inch strip out of the white construction paper.

Activity: Ask your children to tell you ways they keep their teeth healthy. Possible responses include: I brush my teeth, I eat healthy foods, I floss my teeth, and I see a dentist. Foster the idea that taking care of their teeth in these ways will keep their baby teeth healthy and strong and will help their permanent teeth grow in that way, too.

Then let the children make Happy Teeth pictures. Give each child one of the smiling lips shapes and a white paper strip. Have the children snip off little pieces of their white strip to make "teeth," and then glue the teeth to the lip shape to make big toothy smiles. Let them take the smiles home to remind them of all the ways they can make their teeth happy.

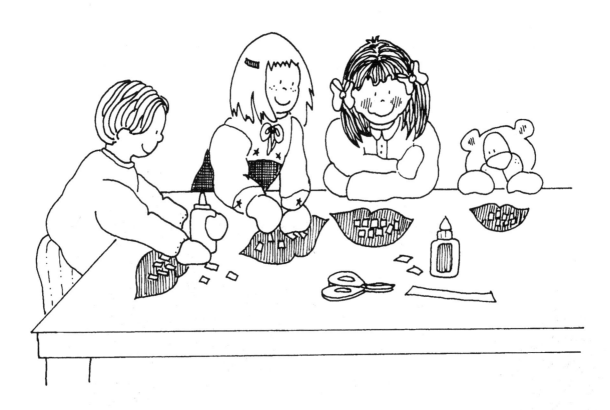

Sun Protection

Help your children learn how to protect themselves from the sun's rays with this Bear Hug.

Materials: Butcher paper; felt tip marker; yellow and orange crayons; scissors.

Preparation: Draw a large sun shape on the butcher paper. Place the paper on a table or on the floor.

Activity: Have your children use the crayons to color in the sun. Talk about the sun while they are coloring. Tell them that the sun is actually a star that is very close to us. It is very bright and very hot. The warmth they feel when they go outside on a sunny day is coming from the sun's rays.

When the children have finished coloring the sun, cut it out and hang it up in the room. Have the children pretend that their paper sun is the real sun. Have them walk all around the room. While they are walking, explain that no matter where they are, the rays from the sun can reach them. Tell them that this is very nice because the rays will keep them warm, but when the sun's rays shine on them for long periods of time, the rays can hurt their eyes and skin.

Ask the children if they know how to protect their eyes and skin from the sun. Possible answers include: wearing hats, putting on sunscreen, wearing sunglasses, and staying indoors in the middle of the day. Help your children remember to put these ideas into action by having sunscreen available, asking the children to bring hats and sunglasses to wear, and staying inside during the brightest part of the day.

Hint: Encourage your children to wear sunscreen by letting them practice putting lotion on a plastic doll.

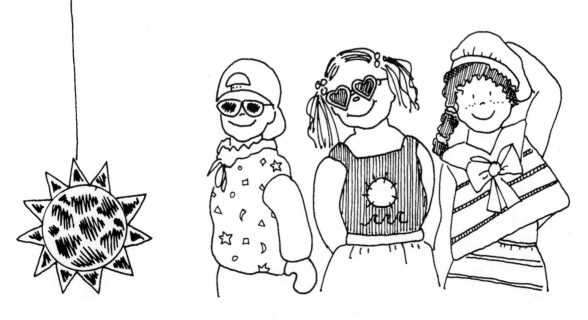

TEACHER RESOURCES

1001 SERIES

These super reference books are filled with just the right solution, prop, or poem to get your projects going. Creative, inexpensive ideas await you!

1001 Teaching Props
The ultimate how-to prop book to plan projects and equip discovery centers. Comprehensive materials index lets you create projects with recyclable materials. 248 pp.
WPH 1501

1001 Teaching Tips
Shortcuts to success for busy teachers on limited budgets. Curriculum, room, and special times tips—even a subject index. 208 pp.
WPH 1502

1001 Rhymes & Fingerplays
A complete language resource for parents and teachers! Rhymes for all occasions, plus poems about self-esteem, families, special needs, and more. 312 pp.
WPH 1503

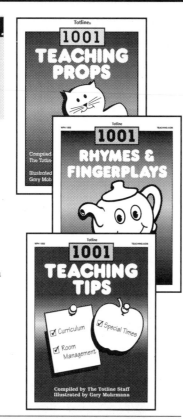

1•2•3 SERIES

These books present simple, hands-on activities that reflect Totline's commitment to providing open-ended, age-appropriate, cooperative, and no-lose experiences for working with preschool children.

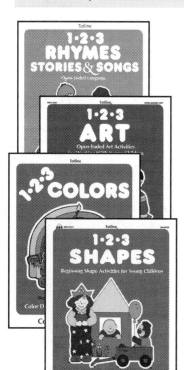

1•2•3 Art *Open-ended Art*
160 pages of art activities emphasize the creative process. All 238 activities use inexpensive, readily available materials. 160 pp.
WPH 0401

1•2•3 Colors
Hundreds of activities for Color Days, including art, learning games, language, science, movement, music, and snacks. 160 pp.
WPH 0403

1•2•3 Books
More than 20 simple concept books to make, including sequences, textures, and weather. 80 pp.
WPH 0406

1•2•3 Murals *Cooperative Art*
More than 50 simple murals to make from children's open-ended art. 80 pp.
WPH 0405

1•2•3 Reading & Writing
250 meaningful and non-threatening activities to develop pre-reading and pre-writing skills. 160 pp.
WPH 0407

BEAR HUGS SERIES

This unique series uses a positive approach for dealing with potential problem times. Great ideas for handling specific group situations. Each 24 pp.

Remembering the Rules
These simple rule reminders are fun and nonthreatening.
WPH 2501

Staying in Line
Make staying in line fun, quiet, and safe.
WPH 2502

Circle Time
Get children interested and involved in circle time.
WPH 2503

Transition Times
Help children smoothly shift focus from one activity to another.
WPH 2504

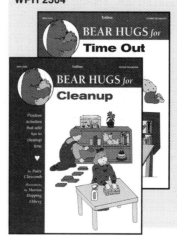

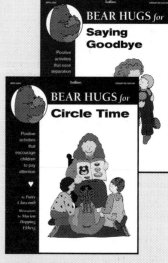

Time Out
Encourage reflective and therapeutic time outs that get results!
WPH 2505

Saying Goodbye
Ease separation anxiety with simple activities and gentle distractions.
WPH 2506

Nap Time
Guide reluctant children into quiet, restful moods.
WPH 2509

Meals and Snacks
Quiet young ones so they can eat without dampening their spirits.
WPH 2507

Cleanup
Encourage cooperation and speedy work with fun cleanup times.
WPH 2508

1•2•3 Rhymes, Stories & Songs *Open-ended Language*
Open-ended rhymes, stories, and songs for young children. 80 pp.
WPH 0408

NEW! 1•2•3 Shapes
Hundreds of activities for exploring the concept of shapes—circles, squares, triangles, rectangles, ovals, diamonds, hearts, and stars. 160 pp.
WPH 0411

1•2•3 Math
Hands-on activities, such as counting, sequencing, and sorting, help develop pre-math skills. 160 pp.
WPH 0409

1•2•3 Science
Develop science skills—observing, estimating, predicting—using ordinary household objects. 160 pp.
WPH 0410

1•2•3 Games *No-Lose Games*
Foster creativity and decision-making with 70 no-lose games for a variety of young ages. 80 pp.
WPH 0402

1•2•3 Puppets
More than 50 simple puppets to make to delight children. 80 pp.
WPH 0404

TEACHING THEMES

BUSY BEES

For Two's and Three's
Day-by-day, hands-on projects and activities are just right for busy little ones.

Busy Bees—FALL
For fall fun and learning, these attention-getting activities include songs, rhymes, snacks, movements, art, and science projects. 136 pp.
WPH 2405

Busy Bees—WINTER
Enchant toddlers through winter with a wealth of seasonal ideas, from movement to art. 136 pp.
WPH 2406

Busy Bees—SPRING
More than 60 age-appropriate activities enhance learning for busy minds and bodies. 136 pp.
WPH 2407

Busy Bees—SUMMER
Encourage toddlers to build, develop, and explore with their senses and turn summer fun into learning. 136 pp.
WPH 2408

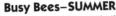
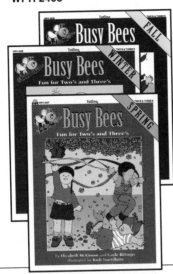

PLAY & LEARN

This creative, hands-on series explores the versatile play and learn opportunities of a familiar object. Perfect for working with young children ages 3 to 8. Each 64 pp.

Play & Learn with Photos
WPH 2303

Play & Learn with Magnets
WPH 2301

Play & Learn with Rubber Stamps
WPH 2302

CELEBRATIONS

Expand on your children's love for celebrations with these ideas for special learning fun.

Small World Celebrations
Multicultural Units • 160 pp.
WPH 0701

Special Day Celebrations
Nontraditional Units • 128 pp.
WPH 0702

Yankee Doodle Birthday Celebrations
Antibias Units • 128 pp.
WPH 0703

Great Big Holiday Celebrations
Traditional Units • 228 pp.
WPH 0704

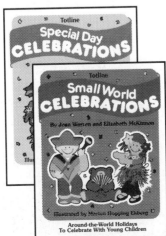
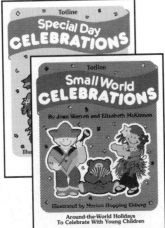

THEME-A-SAURUS

Capture special teaching moments with instant theme ideas that cover around-the-curriculum activities.

Theme-A-Saurus
50 teaching themes—from Apples to Zebras—plus 600 fun and educational activity ideas. 280 pp.
WPH 1001

Theme-A-Saurus II
Sixty more teaching units—from Ants to Zippers—for hands-on learning experiences. 280 pp.
WPH 1002

Toddler Theme-A-Saurus
Sixty teaching themes combine safe, appropriate materials with creative activity ideas. 280 pp.
WPH 1003

Alphabet Theme-A-Saurus
From A to Z—26 giant letter recognition units filled with hands-on activities introduce young children to the *ABC's*. 280 pp.
WPH 1004

Nursery Rhyme Theme-A-Saurus
Capture the interest children have for nursery rhymes and extend it into learning. 160 pp.
WPH 1005

Storytime Theme-A-Saurus
Flannelboard patterns accompany 12 storytime favorites, plus hands-on activities and songs. 160 pp.
WPH 1006

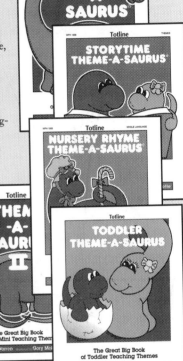

EXPLORING SERIES

Environments
Selected environments become very real places in this book series that encourages exploration. Hands-on activities emphasize all the curriculum areas. Each book begins with the "known" and lets the curriculum expand as far as children's interests can stretch.

Exploring Sand and the Desert
WPH 1801

Exploring Water and the Ocean
WPH 1802

Exploring Wood and the Forest
WPH 1803

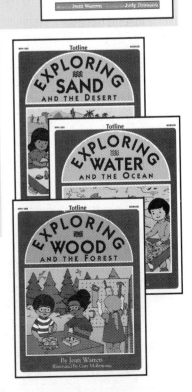

Instant Hands-on Ideas!

FREE sample newsletters available!

Totline® Newsletter

This newsletter offers creative hands-on activities that are designed to be challenging for children ages 2 to 6, yet easy for teachers and parents to do. Minimal preparation time is needed to make maximum use of common, inexpensive materials. Each bimonthly issue includes • seasonal fun • learning games • open-ended art • music and movement • language activities • science fun • reproducible teaching aids • reproducible parent-flyer pages and • Good Earth (environmental awareness) activities. *Totline Newsletter* is perfect for use with an antibias curriculum or to emphasize antibias values in a home environment.

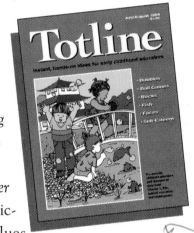

Super Snack News

This newsletter is designed to be reproduced!

With each subscription you are permitted to make up to 200 copies per issue! They make great handouts to parents. Inside this monthly, four-page newsletter are healthy recipes and nutrition tips, plus related songs and activities for young children. Also provided are category guidelines for the CACFP reimbursement program. Sharing *Super Snack News* is a wonderful way to help promote quality childcare.

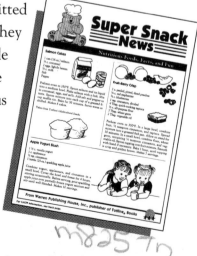

To receive your FREE copy of either Totline Newsletter or Super Snack News, call 1-800-773-7240.